AF124345

12 STEPS TO venus

Isaac Walker

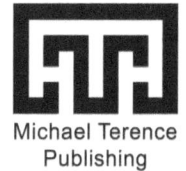
Michael Terence Publishing

First published in paperback by
Michael Terence Publishing in 2019
www.mtp.agency

Copyright © 2019 Isaac Walker

Isaac Walker has asserted his right to be identified as the
author of this work in accordance with the
Copyright, Designs and Patents Act 1988

ISBN 9781913289072

All rights reserved. No part of this publication may be reproduced, stored
in a retrieval system, or transmitted, in any form or by any means,
electronic, mechanical, photocopying, recording or otherwise, without the
prior permission of the publishers

Cover image
Copyright © Evgeniya Porechenskaya

Cover design
Copyright © 2019 Michael Terence Publishing

12 STEPS TO VENUS

Isaac Walker

CONTENTS

PREFACE 1

CHAPTER 1 - CUT TO THE CHASE 5

CHAPTER 2 - THINK OUTSIDE THE BOX 11

CHAPTER 3 - ARTIFICIAL INTELLIGENCE 20

CHAPTER 4 - NO PAIN NO GAIN 30

CHAPTER 5 - MIND OVER MATTER 34

CHAPTER 6 - ESTABLISH THE ROLE 40

CHAPTER 7 - CONNECTION IS KEY 44

CHAPTER 8 - TAKE CONTROL 49

CHAPTER 9 - SEIZE THE MOMENT 56

CHAPTER 10 - SELF INDULGE 60

CHAPTER 11 - PAY CLOSE ATTENTION 65

CHAPTER 12 - 'MAN UP' 72

PREFACE

I think any young child called 'ugly' by his own mother would develop a complex, and this wasn't helped during my teenage years when my face looked more like the moon's surface than that of a fresh-faced teenager. By the time I was 15 most of my friend's had lost their virginity, so the pressure was certainly on for me to lose mine; but with the ever-depleting confidence and the ever-increasing number of rejections, I resorted to using money acquired on my 16th birthday to pay a prostitute for sex. I had finally done it...

Fast forward three years and my continued lack of confidence propelled me towards a life of drugs. Pre-rolled spliffs and lines of cocaine were often part of a daily routine, until one day, I mistakenly snorted Catsan cat litter, while looking for crumbs of cocaine on the floor. I had reached a new low. With no job, no prospects and absolutely no confidence, I decided to join The Prince's Trust's 12-week self-development programme, which breathed new life into a seemingly dead sense of living. Following this experience, I managed to obtain a voluntary role within a youth organisation, and it was during this time I met a man named Ray Austin (mentioned in this book).

Slowly but surely my confidence grew, and as the confidence grew, so too did my success with women. However, my new-found confidence did not make me immune from this thing called life, and it wasn't long before I was the victim of a failed relationship in which my ex-girlfriend left me for another man. This led me towards a downward spiral and subsequent depression. At the time I thought it would be a brilliant idea to resume my drug habit of daily pre-rolled spliffs and lines of cocaine. For the next year or so my life revolved around my PlayStation, bedroom door and the local jobcentre.

I eventually stopped my drug use and sought a job supporting vulnerable people. I began working for the YMCA before working as an Outreach Floating Support Worker. During my time working as an Outreach Floating Support Worker I was introduced to online dating by a colleague, and it was through this experience I began to look into patterns of behaviour displayed by women.

Through failed dates, advice given as well as my own observations I began to become more successful in terms of dating. I shared my experiences with colleagues, and a colleague of mine kept telling me to write a book, as many of the experiences I had shared had helped him with his own dating experiences, but I didn't quite have the belief or the confidence to write a book.

This is all new territory for me but I felt compelled to write this book for two main reasons. 1) To assist men who would normally lack confidence to approach women 2) To provide men with tools I personally have found useful when engaging with women.

The chapters within this book are short, but it does contain universal thoughts and ideas, about today's dating world. The book also contains some strong language and is written in a way to provoke further thought, and where possible, further discussion. The methods mentioned within this book are proven, and they do work. I, therefore, encourage each reader to try them for themselves.

CHAPTER 1 - CUT TO THE CHASE

We've all heard the saying, 'Women are from Mars and Men are from Venus' or whichever way round it goes, and to some extent I think it's true, not in the literal sense but we both find it extremely difficult to understand each other. However, I think the most important thing is first to understand yourself, and what makes you tick as an individual, before attempting to do that with anybody else. Truth of the matter is, we will never ever really get the full picture when it comes to our sexual counterpart and vice versa, but whoever said we had to? People often spend weeks, months, or even years trying to get to know someone but the fact remains, a person will only show you what they want you to see. Therefore, know yourself and embrace the person you are, regardless.

The cliché saying is 'if you don't accept yourself for who you are, then nobody else will'. This isn't necessarily true in my opinion but in terms of the subject matter, it means you've lost your way before you've even got started. I often compare dating to the job application process. You show interest (initial job application form), if the interest is reciprocated you move on to stage 2 (chatting/getting to know each other), if all goes well there, you'll get shortlisted to stage 3 (exchanging of contact details). This stage is crucial, because it's here that the woman will narrow her candidates down to one or two, from the three she has probably shortlisted to this stage. If successful, you get to the final stage (Date), and it's only until your objective is met that you can consider yourself successful throughout the selection (dating) process.

So, what is your objective? What is it you really want? Do you just want sex? Do you want companionship, or do you want a long-lasting relationship that will last beyond a couple of months? There is no point convincing anybody else of your intentions, if you haven't convinced yourself. As long as you know what you want that's all that really matters. The rest will follow. Supposing you just want sex, do you want what I call a 'splash and dash?' (one off night of passion), a friend with those extra benefits, or a triple F (Fuck Friend Forever)? Once you've decided what you want, you need to execute your intentions carefully. I firmly believe a man can get what he wants from a woman, but he must have 'game', and fully engage the woman. The game itself is simple: 'treat the woman like a lady unless otherwise stated'. This means unless a woman wants to be treated like a piece of shit, treat her like a lady. Operation 'get in her knickers' doesn't just stop there. As a man you have to take charge. When I say this, I don't mean you be the owner, and she be the bitch on the lead, although that might work well in a different scenario, but exert yourself, and be firm. For example, a common question when on a date is: "Where shall we sit?" This shouldn't be up for any negotiation. So many times, men have made the vital mistake of saying: "I don't mind it's up to you". I don't care what any woman from Venus says, they all, yes all, subconsciously or consciously, want a man who takes control, because deep down I believe most women want that sense of stability and security, as well as to feel protected. Now if you're buckling under the weight of indecisiveness, do you think it will show you as a man who can take control? Make a decision, be firm and stick to it! For those who are not so comfortable with this I would suggest you do the following: if you are going to a bar and you really are unsure of where to sit, calmly ask the lady what she would like to drink and casually walk towards the bar. As you do this, tell the woman to find a place to sit, while you order the drinks. Not only are you showing your gentlemanly behaviour by getting the 1st orders, but it shows, in a subtle but effective way, that you can take control, but more importantly it shows your authoritative edge.

While the man has the capabilities to unlock the gateway to a woman's vagina, she will always hold the key, and for this reason it is paramount that the man understands that the woman will always hold the power. In other words, if the woman doesn't want to have sex with you, it simply won't happen. It really is as simple as that. Therefore, you must empower the woman into believing she's in control, and that you're not just taking advantage of her. Women generally don't like to feel cheap, so don't make her feel that way. One simple way you can make the woman feel empowered is to approach her and the date with no expectations. This not only takes the pressure off you but also the woman. It also allows you to approach the date with an open mind and allows each of you to simply go with the flow and enjoy the experience. Another way you can empower the woman is to simply tell her she's in control. Make her know that you know, that without her say so, nothing will happen. It shows that you understand her and you've given her the sense of empowerment, which normally helps towards sealing the deal by the end of the evening, but if that doesn't happen you can almost guarantee it will pave the way towards a second date.

Dr Sai, co-author with Dr Ogi Ogas of "A Billion Wicked Thoughts –What the Internet tells us about Sexual Relationships" said that the male sexual brain is like a toggle switch, all he needs is a visual cue to get aroused. The woman's sexual brain, however, is like the cock pit of a fighter jet plane, full of sensitive equipment. Her actual brain acts like a detective, trying to obtain as much information as possible before deciding whether the man is worth her attention. Therefore, it is important to understand that while appearance or looks generally play a key role in attraction, they are not fundamental! Well, not for all women anyway. With this in mind, it's important that you adhere to what I call the three Cs: confidence; calmness and consideration. Be confident within yourself and who you are. Don't try to be someone you're not. Be you, stay true and if it's meant to be, shit will go down! It's also important to be calm. A clear mind never fails and the ability to stay calm also shows you can handle pressure. It will help to keep the cortisol levels down and will allow you to fully embrace the experience. After all, even failed dates are all part of the learning process. Consideration is almost a forgotten art these days. We're so engrossed in soothing our own needs that we often forget the needs of our significant other. This attribute shows that you are thoughtful and allows room for acceptance. I'm not saying that this will guarantee you a night, or many nights of passion, but I strongly believe that it will provide you with the added ammunition needed to execute your intentions, if it's just sex you're after.

As mentioned previously, the woman will always be the Gatekeeper towards her own body, but the man can manipulate her to gain access. As a man, we are seen in society as the stronger of the two sexes. Thus, we should apply this in the dating arena. A woman will always try, where possible to push the boundaries and see what she can and what she can't get away with. As a result, you will need to stamp your authority and clearly show from the off what you will and what you won't accept. In today's society it is fair to say that women will date multiple men, or even sleep with them, until they get what they want, which is generally that Prince Charming who will sweep her off her feet. This doesn't go for all women of course, but for the large majority of women I have encountered this is generally the case. Therefore, it is conceivable that a woman may well be unlocking the gateway to her sacred crown jewel to another man, while you take the time and effort to get to know her.

This can be a tricky position to be in, because nobody likes to play 2nd, 3rd or 4th fiddle to anyone, especially when you're taking the time and effort to capture her full attention. With that said, you will need to establish whether the time and effort is worth your while. One way you can assess this is to ascertain what it is you truly want from the woman. Do you want to explore the possibility of having a long-lasting relationship or do you want just sex?

If the latter applies, then it is worth assessing her engagement with you. Does she respond in a timely manner? Does she take an interest in getting to know you? Is she receptive to the idea of meeting up? If the answer is no to any of these questions, then chances are she's not worth the hassle. After all there are 24 hours in a day, 60 minutes within each hour and 60 seconds within each minute. The average working day consists of 8 hours. Generally speaking, it takes approximately one and half minutes to write a text message, so I am of the opinion that, if someone fails to respond or they ignore you stating: "I've been too busy" chances are they're not that interested. Same result applies if a woman shows little or no interest in you, nor the prospect of meeting up. On the flip side, if she is showing interest, then it could be that she sees potential in taking things beyond the confines of the bedroom and would like to explore whether or not you are that Prince Charming. However, be under no illusion and think that you are the only man she is expressing this to. Therefore, it is essential that you stand out from the rest.

CHAPTER 2 - THINK OUTSIDE THE BOX

Let's face it the competition for us Men is fierce, and therefore it's easy to understand why women are so ruthless when it comes to diverting their attention elsewhere. Men are somewhat disposable these days, just another number in a pool swarming with infinite hopefuls. So how does one reign supreme amongst the stiff competition? I think it is essential that you find your USP (Unique Selling Point). As sad and as absurd as it may sound, this is what we men have to resort to. How else can one stand out from the rest? Think about it: a woman will get approached several times a day by several different men, and chances are if each of those men is coming up with the same old boring approach, the woman will simply get fed up. In order for you to understand where I'm going with this, think of a time when you've seen a woman that has you gasping for breath. You are feeling reasonably confident and you're in a rampant mood. You take due care and attention when approaching, and you get blasted faster than you can break wind. At that moment, you're thinking what the hell just happened? Well chances are you were probably the 9th or 10th guy to have approached her that day; and it's also likely that you used the same approach as the guys that fell victim to her rejection before you. Therefore, it is so important that you really try to stand out from the rest. From a personal point of view my USP was to go Gym and build muscle long before the 'Gym craze' took London by storm. When I first became married to the Gym, hardly any of the guys I knew were training. Which meant by the time summer of 2009 came about, I had women tripping over their wedges, stilettos and high-top trainers. I became a novelty that soothed their curiosity of being with a Muscular guy, which suited me just fine, because after the number of anabolic steroids and additional testosterone I had injected into my body, I was like a walking Dildo. I am not suggesting that you take the same drastic approach as I did, but you have to make yourself stand out. It could be in your appearance or the way in which you approach women, which leads me nicely on to my next point: 'The Approach'.

Nobody likes to be rejected, especially in full view of other people, but there are occasions when we see a woman that we like, that we may have to take that risk. I myself have suffered countless rejections in my time, some of which have left me begging for the ground to open up wide and gobble me up, but I know I am not alone there. Through this experience, I began to think of the ways in which I could approach women, whilst limiting the possibility of being rejected in front of other people. One answer I came up with was not to approach women in public - full stop. However, that for me was a 'no go' area as this only limited the possibilities of getting to meet/know a woman I desired. I then began to think of all the possible scenarios in which you would need to speak with a stranger, without the risk of their thinking you're a complete weirdo. Suddenly I had a lightbulb moment and thought... Asking for directions! Not knowing where you are going and asking for directions is completely normal, but also acts as a perfect excuse to approach any woman that has you drooling over them. I put this to the test when on a tube journey to Paddington.

I remember being on the tube when a tall Amazonian blonde, standing at around 5ft 11, with a sun-kissed golden tan, came and sat opposite me. She was wearing a black skirt that came up just above her knees, which were perfect for showing off her well-developed legs, which I must add appeared smooth and very well kept. Her calves were shaped like diamonds and were thick, just how I like them. Funnily enough she looked exactly like a woman I had tried to approach 2 months' before. I remember looking at her at every given opportunity, whilst trying to avoid being blatantly obvious. We caught each other's eye a few times but at no point did I have the balls to approach her. As the train went from station to station, I was carefully trying to plan my next move. I thought of all the different possible scenarios in which I could approach her, which subsequently led to an internal dialogue. I asked myself: shall I get off at the same stop as her even if her stop is before or after mine? Shall I smile at her the next time she catches my eye? Shall I wink at her instead? Then I thought "fuck it!" what will be will be. "The next station is Paddington" announced the female voice over the TFL Tannoy. At that point "fuck it" soon turned to "oh shit" but fortunately she got off at the same stop as me. By this time my heart was beating at a rate that far exceeded the average heartbeat, and my mouth was so dry anyone would think I had returned from the wilderness within the Sahara Desert, but with anxiety gathering momentum, I used this to my advantage to appear authentic. "Excuse me, do you know how to get to Gloucester Road?" I asked anxiously. I knew exactly how to get to Gloucester Road, but she didn't know that, and she wasn't supposed to, as I needed the perfect excuse to approach her. "Yes" she responded, revealing her pearl white teeth through her welcoming smile. She kindly told me exactly how to get to where I knew already. I responded by profusely thanking her and asked if I could show my appreciation by taking her for a drink? She seemed pleasantly surprised and said yes. We exchanged numbers and I met her a week later and the rest is history.

There were a few things I considered when adopting this approach. 1) Know where you are going, or have a rough idea where you are going, beforehand. For instance, if the woman you wish to approach is going in a similar direction to the one you already know, it provides you with the perfect excuse to follow her, with the intention of asking her where you need to go, rather than have an extra few minutes to perv and seem like a weirdo sexual predator stalking her. 2) There is every possibility somebody else, other than the woman you want, may offer to give directions. Therefore, ensure you are clear as to whom you are seeking directions from. In other words, be direct and go straight to the woman, rather than make it seem as though you are openly asking for directions. 3) The woman may not know how you will need to get to your destination, which means the line: "Can I show my appreciation by taking you for a drink" is redundant. However, if you are confident enough you may still wish to engage the woman in a conversation in the hope you will obtain her contact number.

As mentioned before nobody likes to be rejected in the face of other people, but I believe FEAR (False Expectations About Reality) will only limit your chances when it comes to women. Having said that, we are human and as humans we are prone to feel anxious, and a sense of fear and uneasiness when faced by an uncomfortable situation, but I think it is better to work within the anxiety, fear and uneasiness, rather than just shy away from them. Do not think of the worst possible scenario but think of the best possible way to deal with the worst possible scenario. For instance, you are on the train and you see a beautiful woman that has the blood flowing to all parts of your anatomy. You are mesmerised, aroused and excited all at the same time and the train is jam packed. Would you take the chance and approach her? Chances are 80 to 85% of the time you won't, and that is me being generous with the percentage scale. Realistically speaking, most men will gaze and end up having to take their coat, or bag to cover up the young man downstairs. Reason being, the majority, if not all, will think of the worst possible outcome, which is getting rejected in front of everybody within the carriage but if we considered my point about finding the best possible way to deal with the worst possible outcome, then you will find that you have nothing to lose every single time. Supposing we could get rejected without anyone finding out? I am sure that would increase the number of individuals willing to take a risk on approaching a woman, when in a crowded environment. So how do I apply this you may ask? Well it is simple. Think Pen and Paper. Now I know we live in an age where technology is far exceeding the traditional means of communication, but a simple pen and a bit of paper is all you actually need.

I can recall sitting and speaking with a colleague of mine, on the way home from work, when a woman caught my eye. My colleague and I were talking about work, obviously, and as we were talking, I could feel my attention being diverted. I don't know what came over me, but I began looking into my bag for a piece of paper and pen, which I eventually found. As my colleague was speaking, I calmly wrote my number along with my name and a message asking the lady to call me. I was subtle about this, as I did not want my colleague to realise what I was doing, so in between nodding and acknowledging what my colleague was saying, I was quietly writing on the piece of paper. I folded the paper and held onto it. When the time came for the woman to get off the train I said: "Excuse me Miss, you dropped something" and then handed her the piece of paper containing my number. She thanked me and got off the train. I never did hear from her, but that isn't the point. The point is my colleague along with everybody else on the train were oblivious to the fact I had made a move. Not even she was privy to the fact I was trying it on until the moment she unfolded the piece of paper and saw my number written on it.

Business cards work the same way, and in my view better to use. There have been countless occasions, when I have been out at an event and I have written "Call me" along with a kiss or smiley face on the back of my business card. Most of the time people think I am just trying to promote my service, and again are oblivious to the fact I am making my intentions known.

In order for us to master the art of dating, we must learn to choose our battles carefully. Even a hungry lioness applies caution when hunting her prey. Therefore, we must carefully consider when is a good time and when isn't a good time to approach a woman. Now for some of you reading this, there never, ever seems to be a good time to approach a woman, which is probably why you may be reading this, but there are times when I firmly believe that we just have to accept defeat and move on. A classic example of this is when you're faced with the 'cock blocking' friend. I never could understand why a woman would go out of her way to hinder a man's chances of approaching her friend, but thinking back to how some of them looked, it's no wonder they allowed themselves to be possessed by the 'Green Eyed Monster'. It's frustrating because you meet a woman, you're getting along really well, and just as you reach a point when you feel you can exchange contact details, her friend comes along and fucks the whole thing up. I can't lie, but if there is ever an occasion when I would consider 'throttling a woman' it's then. This face off with the cock blocking friend has happened to me on more than one occasion, which is why I have a golden rule: never take the initiative to approach a woman when she's with a friend. I say this with conviction and because of two main reasons. 1) She's probably not that interested anyway, and generally speaking, women who are with their friends are focused on spending that time with them. 2) Her friend will always prevail, so even if she did have the intention of getting to know you, she probably won't if her friend doesn't approve. Of course, this isn't always the case, but from my experience this is the conclusion I have come to.

I think approaching a woman when she is with two other friends may be a safer option. Again, from my experience, the woman you are approaching acts as a focal point for her friends to talk and gossip about. This plays right into your hands, because the friends will generally allow the process to unfold whilst they will have each other as company to talk to, and possibly make fun of the friend as you are approaching her. This is a case-by-case scenario, but I can only go by what's worked for me and my experience.

Another 'no go' for me is approaching women during a night out on a Friday/Saturday evening. Most people are out over the weekend and most men see this as the perfect opportunity to approach women, but sadly this is self-esteem suicide. The large majority of men will get rejected, which then propels them to get into a 'punch up', get thrown out of a club/bar, visit their local Kebab shop, vomit on the way home, struggle to get their key into the front door and finish the night off with their right hand. Don't get me wrong I am not suggesting for one moment that it is not possible to get a woman, when on a night out during the weekend, but you're probably better off diverting your attention away from the weekend hype, and focus it towards a quiet wine bar in the city on a Tuesday or Wednesday evening after work. Now this does depend on the type of woman you tend to go for, as most, if not all, who visit a local bar after work on a weekday are working professionals, ranging from mid 30s to early 50s, or those who are lonely and seeking that special person to snuggle up with and watch meaningless shit on TV. Generally speaking, these kinds of women are too focused and career driven to turn their attentions towards establishing a relationship. More often than not, they tend to prefer the no strings approach. That is not to say that the woman will engage or have sex with any man that approaches her, but it does cut out a good percentage of the red-blooded male competitors.

CHAPTER 3 - ARTIFICIAL INTELLIGENCE

While the approaches I have discussed are tried and tested methods, we have reached an age now in which online dating seems to be the only realistic way of meeting somebody. I guess it's far easier to swipe, click and wink than it is to pluck up the courage to approach someone face to face; but as the old saying goes, "If you can't beat them join them", so when entering the world of online dating it is important to note that first impressions are generally lasting impressions, and therefore crucial that you create a profile that captures the attention of the woman. Most men attempt to solve this problem by uploading numerous topless pictures, either of them in the gym or at home in front of their bathroom mirror, flexing their arms or tensing their torso. For the superficial types, this works a treat, but if you are attempting to attract a woman with substance and decorum this is a fatal mistake, and this is because of two main reasons. 1) The topless picture does not leave anything for the imagination, which women thrive on. 2) This leads the woman into believing you only want one thing (sex) and as stated in an earlier chapter, women generally do not like to feel cheap.

Just remember, first impressions are lasting impressions, so refrain from uploading the half-naked selfies, and upload pictures of you within a social setting. For example, pictures of you out in a bar with friends, or pictures of you on holiday, or at an event will provoke the woman into wanting to find out more as it will show you as a man who is socially adaptable, but more importantly someone who appears to be fun. Ever heard Cyndi Lauper's 'Girl's Just Wanna Have Fun?' Well that just about sums our Female counterparts up. Women generally just want to have fun and the more fun and outgoing you appear to the woman, the more likely it is you will be able to capture her attention, but her attention span goes beyond the uploaded pictures. Women have a tendency to pay close attention to detail, especially when coming across a profile on a dating website. Therefore, you shouldn't be surprised if I told you she will probably read your profile. With this in mind, refrain from using colloquial terms such as: 'wots up', 'ello babe' and 'that's kool' to name a few. Ensure your grammar game is on point and you check for spelling errors too. For the more sophisticated types, these errors (spelling and grammar) are a major turn off, so please do bear this in mind.

I believe the content on your profile is paramount, and I would go as far as to say that it is slightly more important than the pictures. Unless you want cheap thrills with a woman who could belong to anybody, I would suggest the following 1) Write a punchy headline which is short, sweet and sums you up in a nutshell. 2) Refrain from writing a mini essay 3) Keep the bio section short and if possible 'tongue in cheek'.

An example: if I had to use three words to describe myself, I'd say: dynamic, easy-going and impulsive. Technically that's four words! Ah well.........I'm what you would call a social butterfly, in that I adapt to suit my surroundings. Some may see this as a personality disorder, but I think this makes me socially adaptable. Believe it or not my mind stretches far beyond my bulging biceps, so if you're after much needed mental stimulation then look no further. Modesty was never my strong point.

As you can see this isn't some long drawn out bio, in which I am using all of the superlatives known to man to describe myself, nor am I expressing my deepest desire to meet the ideal woman. I am using humour in a jovial way to describe the person I am, whilst ensuring that I do not give too much away. By doing this, it puts the woman into inquisitive mode, and therefore provokes her into getting in touch.

It is one thing setting up a profile which captures the attention of a woman, but it is another thing contacting a woman with a message that goes beyond the words "Hi, how are you?" Unfortunately, most men do not look beyond the uploaded pictures displayed on the woman's profile, and while this will be acceptable for the man who is blessed with God-given good looks, for the large majority this is a costly mistake. You can save yourself time and energy by first reading the profile. I say this because I have made the mistake of messaging a woman, and then later left wondering why she hasn't been in touch, only to discover that it clearly stated on her profile that she does not go for men of my ethnic origin, or she will only consider dates with men within a 5-mile radius. Having said that, it is also useful to read her profile to get an overview of what she is seeking but also to get a sense of the type of woman she could be. When doing this, I would use a line within her profile as an opening line for my message. For example, if she states Lady seeking her Prince Charming, I would say something along the lines of: "How many Frogs have you had to kiss until now?" My name's Ike, why don't you come by and say hi? This approach hasn't always got me a response, but that's ok because I'm not going to be to everyone's taste.

During the initial stages of online conversation, it is important to keep the woman engaged. This is always a difficult task to achieve, especially when there's another man lurking in the background ready to pounce, but as long as you keep the spotlight firmly on the woman, whilst keeping the interaction light hearted and not too intense, then you should be ok. I think it is worth pointing out, unless the woman asks you a question, do not be quick to give her any information. I believe it is more effective if you keep the spotlight on her and find out as much as you possibly can, without her feeling interrogated. If she is genuinely interested, then she will naturally ask you questions anyway.

Depending on how the interaction goes will determine when I decide to ask for her number. For example, if there is a good rapport and it is clear she is interested, then I would message quite early on something along the lines of: "How do you feel about exchanging numbers?" By asking in this way it does not make her feel pressured, but rather reinforces the fact she is in control. I personally can count on one hand the number of women that have refused to give me their number by my asking this way, and even if they have refused, they will respond by saying: "I would like to get to know you more" or "I'm sorry I think it's too soon...."Either way you're still leaving yourself with a chance.

Generally speaking, after the online phase of contact you will move onto the phone stage (as just explained). During this stage, if the contact is going well, it is highly likely she will inform you that she has left the dating site/app but do not be convinced by this. Ask yourself: why would a woman delete her profile and focus all her efforts on someone she hasn't even met? Don't get me wrong, there are a select few who still maintain a level of honesty and respect, who still long and hope for that Knight in shining Armour to sweep her off her feet, and will adopt this kind of approach if necessary, but this is normally after a date has taken place. For the large majority, they will convince you that they have left the dating site/app in the hope of one of two outcomes: 1) The man does not see her as a cheap slag who has loads of men on the go. 2) She is hopeful the man will follow suit and delete his profile and focus all his attention on her. Fact of the matter is women generally do not like to feel any sense of guilt and will sway this feeling by either avoidance - convincing you her profile is deleted, or diversion - giving you the sense of feeling guilty because she's deleted her profile and you still have yours. While the woman's disclosure regarding her profile is plausible, it is unlikely for the reasons I have stated.

I guess the obvious solution to the topic regarding details of the woman's profile status is to check but women, unlike their male counterparts, cover their tracks. Women can be very cunning and I will expose exactly what they do, while they try to convince you they have permanently deleted their profile. For this I am going to use 'Plenty Of Freaks'- I mean 'Plenty Of Fish'- as an example, as it is the most recognised of all the dating sites/apps. Firstly, the woman will block you from contacting her, as this will remove all correspondence, giving you the impression that she has disappeared into thin air. Secondly, she will hide her profile to ensure that she does not show up in any of the searches on the POF app, again giving the impression that she is no longer there. As stated a moment ago, women seek one of two outcomes as a result; and while the ultimate goal is to achieve whatever it is you set out to achieve within the dating context, it is important to be aware of the things I have just mentioned.

As with most things we experience in life, there are ups and downs, peaks and troughs, highs and lows, good spells and bad spells and the online dating scene is no different. So, there will be occasions in which you're actively receiving messages and responses and other times in which you're getting blanked left, right and centre. When the latter happens, I resort to an old trick. I simply hide my profile for a week or so, and then I unhide it. The reason I do this is because I will show as a recent new member. Therefore, if a newbie comes along and joins the online world of dating, I will show up when they conduct searches, which means I am on display to a wider range of women. Another thing that can help you along the 'blankety blank cheque book and pen moment' is to re-vamp your profile. New pictures, new bio and a brand-new profile username should help do the trick.

There is a large number of online dating websites and apps and I would certainly recommend joining the free ones to help whet the appetite. Free sites such as Plenty OF Fish (POF) and Tinder seem to be good, although you do have to be careful on sites such as POF. I had an incident once when a woman messaged me expressing an interest. At first, I thought it was too good to be true, and generally speaking it often is, but after we exchanged contact details and she sent me pictures via WhatsApp, I was convinced she was genuine. During our interactions on WhatsApp, she informed me that she is a qualified masseuse and she specialises in deep tissue Swedish massages. Me being me, I made a joke and asked "will that include a happy ending?" to which she responded "my normal fee for an hour is £70 but for you I can do it for £50." I thought she was taking the piss, but she was dead serious. Turns out the woman was a hooker, who was using POF to get new clients. I guess for those who think economically, £50 is a bargain, considering the fact you'll spend far more than that on a night out with a date, but I thrive on the chase, so to have something handed to me on a plate like that didn't appeal. Moreover, a woman should not be treated like a 'slab of meat'.

Through the online dating experience, I have come to realise that there are different types of women, who access different types of online dating sites. The rule of thumb is that all the women that access these sites want to find a man they can 'settle down' with, but the way in which they go about it is different. For instance, women who are actively on sites such as Tinder want sex first and a decent guy after. These women tend to fuck their way through the site, while maintaining a desire to find the 'right one'. I accept that this is a broad and generalised comment, but other than pictures, there really is nothing else a woman can go by. So, if her perception of the man is purely based upon his physical appearance, then it is likely her objective to get with a man will be driven by sex. The same can almost be said about those who access Plenty Of Fish. These women tend to have a stronger desire to meet the right man but they too like a fair bit of nookie. Then there are sites such as Match.com and E Harmony. The sites which are designed for the hardcore, genuine long-term seeker. You are more inclined to find a woman willing to wait 2 months before you share a kiss, than a woman willing to rip your shirt open after a few hours. Due to the membership fees, which add value and subsequent quality to the respective sites, you are likely to find women who are seeking their Knight in Shining Armour, unlike those on POF and Tinder willing to pick up Knights in their tin foil armour. Of course, the sites/apps I have just mentioned are the main ones which individuals use, but there are others such as Badoo and SKOUT. These are blatant 'hook up' sites in which the primary objective is sex. There have been a fair few instances, in which I have messaged a woman in the morning and by the evening of the same day of initial contact, I have managed to find my way towards her bedroom. While these are deemed 'hook up' sites, there is an etiquette one needs to follow, and it does not involve you pulling your trousers down to your ankles, exposing your 'dinky winky', taking a snapshot and sending it as a message along with the caption "Hi, do you fancy a chat?" For those who are prone to 'willy flashing' I would strongly suggest you refrain from doing this, as it will only get you reported and potentially banned from the site. Remember, even a cheap whore does not like to feel like she is one, so don't treat her that way!! Maintain class, respect and dignity, even if it is within the bizarre and wonderful world of online dating.

It is worth noting that within the sites I have just mentioned, there are different categories of women. For example, there is the type of woman you wouldn't be caught dead walking on the street with. These women are purely there for sexual purposes and you couldn't care less about them or their feelings. Then there are the women who you wouldn't mind being seen in public with, but you don't want your peers to know you have any dealings with them; these women are considered to be the 'dirty little secret'. You also have the woman who you like, but not enough to commit long term to and tend to keep her dangling on a long piece of string. Then you have the women that will have you jumping through hoops just to capture her attention, let alone anything else. Generally speaking, it doesn't take a rocket scientist to figure out that your intentions towards a woman are based on your behaviour and while you may think the woman is oblivious to this, I can assure you that she is more clued up than you think. A woman will go along with whatever dynamic you create, as long as it is conducive towards fulfilling her needs, but the moment she feels that it no longer serves a purpose, then she will dis-engage. However, providing you treat the woman with respect, the disengagement process will follow three main stages: the break- up or stopping of whatever you had going on; the act or the pursuit of something to take their mind off you and the time you spent together; and then there's the time to reflect. The latter is key, as it is during this phase the woman will review whether she's done the right thing, and if you've treated her with a level of respect then there is always a possibility you can reignite that flame.

CHAPTER 4 - NO PAIN NO GAIN

Women as some of you may know are fickle creatures, and their responses are based upon their mood. So, if a woman is generally pissed off with all living men, the chances are she will show little compassion or remorse when 'blowing you out'. Despite the sheer brutality of her rejection there will be no subtlety about the way she delivers it. In fact, some women can be extremely cold hearted when rejecting a man's advances, but try not to take this personally, as I believe there's always an underlying reason/issue when a person behaves like a complete 'Dickhead'. This is generally a projection of them and the person they are, rather than you. I mention this because it's important to be observant and gauge the mood of the woman before even attempting to make an approach. I remember walking down the street in my local area, when I saw a tall, Amazonian blonde standing at around 5ft 11. Sound familiar? Well it should, because this was the exact same woman I asked for directions, when on the tube to Paddington Station. On this occasion, when I approached her, she took one look up and another look down, rolled her eyes, completely ignored me and walked on. She had absolutely no interest in me whatsoever, so much so I felt like the brown smelly stuff people often get at the bottom of their shoes. Having said that, if I had applied the same caution as to the hungry lioness, I could have saved myself the embarrassment, but this is ironic considering the fact I approached the same woman approximately 2 months later and ended up getting her number amongst other things. I put this down to her fickle nature, and the fact she was probably bombarded with so many men approaching her, that she probably didn't even remember who I was. In essence, the point I am trying to make here is that you should apply caution before approaching the woman. Look out for clues that suggest the mood she is in, and If you get a negative vibe don't approach her. However, if you do and she rejects you, don't instantly think it's because of you. It could be that you've caught her on a bad day. Having said that, if you catch her on a different day dust yourself off and try again.

Rejection can have a long lasting and damaging effect on one's confidence and self- esteem. According to some studies, our brain responds to rejection the same way it responds to physical pain, which can go some way to explaining why rejection can hurt so bad. From my early teens right up until my mid-20s, I had very low confidence when it came to women. This was a direct result of countless knock backs and rejection from a vast array of women I had approached. My confidence was so low that I would be a nervous wreck, if I came into close proximity with a woman I found attractive. I would always look away or look down, and this was all due to the rejection I had suffered at the hands of women. It wasn't until a man by the name of Ray Austin sat me down in a KFC store in Kingsland Road, Dalston and told me about the Flavoured Crisp Analogy. According to Ray we are like assorted flavoured crisps. Some might like Salt & Vinegar flavoured crisps, whilst others may like Ready Salted, Prawn Cocktail or Cheese and Onion flavoured crisps. While some may have a favourite, we simply cannot be to everyone's taste. Ever since then I have applied the same line of thinking with women. Some will like me, and some simply will not, but that's ok because I know for every woman who doesn't like me, there will be at the very least one who does. I think it is essential to maintain this line of thinking, because the last thing you want is to doubt the person you are and get sucked into a pool of self-pity. Therefore, never allow the threat of rejection to deter you, and definitely do not fall victim to the damage it could potentially do to your confidence and self-esteem. You are who you are and if the woman you're approaching doesn't want you, rest assure another one will. This does not mean you undertake a 'scatter gun' approach in which you try it on with ten different women, in the hope at least one will show interest, because If you try it on with ten different women and all ten reject you, it will do no favours for your confidence or self-esteem. However, it is important that you maintain the hunger to keep searching when the opportunity presents itself.

The searching process, if you haven't gathered already, can be tedious and exhausting. A substantial amount of time can be taken throughout this stage, with plenty of effort made with minimal results. From a personal stand point, I have always found the summer months better in terms of searching. Generally speaking, individuals seem happier, more receptive and tolerant. Women also have an increased interest in sex during this time of year. Some studies have suggested that sunlight has been shown to have an association with serotonin, the neurotransmitter which is key towards we human's feeling pleasure. Therefore, it's no wonder a woman will seek to leave her boyfriend high and dry, so she can get her fuck on during the summer months. Contrary to this, winter is the time when we all want to keep warm, and women generally want someone to snuggle up to. Therefore, women will generally tend to settle down during this period, and seek a long-term partner. So, if you want no strings attached fun, then you're probably better off conducting your search during the summer. For some, this is considered 'hunting season', but if you seek something more sustainable, then you will probably have better luck during the winter.

CHAPTER 5 - MIND OVER MATTER

Whilst we men are viewed by women as sexual assassins, our sexual counterparts are psychological fiends, who continuously 'head fuck' us at will. Funny thing is half of the time they don't even understand what's going on in their own heads, let alone ours. What makes it worse is they somehow engage us in this mental sideshow, filled with somersaults and backflips conjured up in a whirlwind of varying thoughts. Truth of the matter is women, in my view are simply confused, or as I like to put it simply complexed. As mentioned earlier a woman's brain works like a detective's, there are so many switches and so many things to consider. Firstly, women are fantasists. They thrive on vivid thoughts and imaginations, and in some cases even get aroused by it. A woman can create the most bizarre, unrealistic scenario in her mind. The deeper embedded it is in her mind the more turned on she seems to get by it. In other words, a woman does not have the need to fulfil her deepest fantasy or make what she thinks of a reality. In order for me to put this into perspective, I want you to think of a time when you have exchanged contact details with a woman, and then spent the next 6 months to a year speaking. The word Catfish might spring to mind, which would be understandable, but I want you to consider the fact that the woman has created the perfect image of you in her mind, and she doesn't want anything to blemish that. If this image appears too good to be true, chances are she will never meet you, and you can kiss goodbye to any hopes of ever meeting her. Reason being, she wants that image she created embedded in her mind. Why? Because they're all mental enthusiasts who have the capacity to get aroused by their own imagination. Simply put, women are fucked in the head.

Every living human being that roams Mother Earth knows women are generally confused. As mentioned before, they have no clue what goes on in their own minds, and they are constantly at loggerheads with themselves. With this in mind it is important to understand that the large majority of women under the age of 40 don't have a clue what they want! So, gentleman please refrain from entering the Mental Sideshow. I am not saying that you cannot find a woman that is compatible for you, but just be prepared to go through the mental bullshit in order to get her. After all, the way the male's brain is wired is totally different to the female brain. We've already established that the man's brain is like a toggle switch and the woman's brain is like the many switches contained within a fighter jet plane but the difference goes beyond that. For example, a man's mind concerns itself with logic (reasoning conducted or assessed according to strict principles of validity) In other words everything appears to be black and white, whereas a woman's mind concerns itself with that infamous grey area.

Yes, the area that does not quite make sense, but we're told to give this thought because not everything is black and white. This line of thinking goes far deeper and goes some way to explain why there are inconsistencies in a woman's behaviour. It's almost as if they use this grey area to justify their fucked-up ways. Having said that, it is still crucial to be aware of this when approaching women. Let's say hypothetically you've recently exchanged contact details with a woman and you're maintaining a good level of communication. She's responsive and engages really well, but for some reason there's a barrier which you cannot seem to break down. She flirts, laughs at your jokes and appears really interested, but you just cannot seem to 'win her over'. Now to the average living human being her behaviour clearly demonstrates a person who is interested and has every intention of taking things further, but according to that grey area the man is a symbol of what the woman desires and not necessarily what she wants. In other words, the man is a representation of what the woman wants, but the man himself is not who she wants. If we apply this in the context of a woman being in a relationship that is hanging on the hinges, it might go some way to show you exactly what I mean. For instance, a woman has reached a point in a relationship whereby she is unsure whether she still wishes to be with the man she's been with for the past 3 plus years. During this process the woman subconsciously makes herself available through her social interactions. She ends up exchanging contact details with a guy within the social set up, not because she necessarily likes the man, but through this interaction she can get a taste of what life without her boyfriend is like. Hence, the man becoming a symbol or representation of what she desires. Fucked up? I couldn't agree more. However, this could play kindly into the man's hands, if he is both patient and persistent, and accepts that he is nothing more than an accessory within the situation the woman finds herself in. Women are fickle remember and it will only be a matter of time until patience and persistence prevail.

Now we have established how the woman's mind kind of works, we should consider ways to deal with it. The easiest option is to back off completely and do a 'Cliff Richard', but there would be no fun in that. Besides, we all have needs and as shown in Maslow's Hierarchy of Needs, love/belonging is pretty high up. So how does a man overcome the weird and fucked up world of a woman's mind? Give them as little as possible. Enigma is a man's secret weapon when dealing with the mind of a woman. It is also your best friend when entering the world of dating. Attraction as we know is subjective and while it plays a significant part in the world of dating, it is not the be all and end all. Let us consider Johnny Depp, Michael Jackson and Prince. Now, each of these men are attractive in their own right, but neither of them can be considered oil paintings in my humble opinion. Of course, some may well disagree, but as mentioned attraction is subjective. Now apart from the obvious (fame, lots of money and legions of fans) the one thing that each of these men has in common is mystery. There is an enigmatic energy that draws women to these men, and I believe that it is because of this, that their magnetic field to draw women is so strong. Ever wondered why the Caped Crusader and the Web Slinging Spider get the women? Or why Dracula manages to seduce women at will? Well it is because of their mysteriousness and their ability to keep as much as possible away from the woman's mind. By doing this you leave the woman a void, which she now must fill. This will result in one of two outcomes. She will either create whatever she can to fill that void, or she will do whatever it takes to get to the bottom of whatever the man is keeping from her. Supposing we take the latter into account. This will play right into the hands of a man wishing to court a woman, simply because she will then engage in as much communication as possible to find out as much as she can. The longer the man withholds the information, the longer she engages. This will also feed into her imagination, which we established can be arousing.

In the dating context, the ability not to give off too much also keeps the woman on her toes. So often, when a man meets a stunning woman, he cannot refrain from telling her how stunning she looks, or how pretty/beautiful he thinks she is. I often ask myself, why would a man tell a woman something she already knows? I mean don't they think many men before them wouldn't have said the same thing? I believe by keeping an air of mystery about your perception of her makes her feel uneasy in a curious sense, especially if she's a Stunner. She will be wondering: why hasn't he mentioned anything about the way I look? Doesn't he find me attractive? Is he playing hard to get? Is he gay? Reason being, it is something she is not accustomed to, and from my experience women are always intrigued by something new and unique. Therefore, keep the woman second guessing as much as possible, but not to the point she thinks you're not interested, after all we men are disposable.

Providing you follow some of the things I have outlined thus far, the time will come when you will take a woman out for a date. The date, as previously mentioned is the final stage of the dating application process, but the process cannot be deemed successful, if you have not achieved what you set out to achieve at the beginning. Therefore, there should be no room for complacency when going on a date.

CHAPTER 6 - ESTABLISH THE ROLE

Women just like men will check their date out. While men tend to do this from the top down, women will do this by looking from the bottom up. In other words, the woman will look at what you have on your feet first, before looking at anything else. Women's love affair with footwear goes far deeper than we care to imagine. In fact, footwear for a woman is a statement within itself, a bit like a watch on a man's wrist, although we tend to disregard such aspects in the dating world, but women are sexual detectives remember, so your footwear will play a key role in influencing her decision. Now I am not suggesting for one moment that you take any hard-earned cash and go buy a pair of Prada's or Giuseppe Zanotti's, but I am suggesting that it is imperative you ensure your footwear is clean and presentable. Failure to comply will almost guarantee a failed date, as the woman will develop an image of you that is careless, possibly unhygienic and poor. Particularly, if you are wearing footwear that has gone well passed its sell by date.

A man may also wish to consider his choice of smell. A man's scent can be a powerful tool when attracting a woman and one that acts like a pheromone. For those who are not familiar with pheromones, this is a chemical substance produced and released into the environment, which triggers a social response in members of the same species. The pheromone chemical is capable of acting like hormones outside of the body, to impact the behaviour of the receiving individual. In layman's terms, your scent can have a powerful influence over the woman's attraction towards you. Now you may be asking yourself what type of fragrance should I consider? To be frank, there is no easy answer when it comes to that question, but what I will say is, it's important to pick a fragrance that is compatible with the natural odour of your skin. Just because an aftershave smells nice, it doesn't necessarily mean that it will smell nice on you. Therefore, take your time, shop around and find the right scent for you.

I am a firm believer that a man should be a gentleman, unless it is absolutely necessary to act like a complete asshole. I say this, because it seems the ability to open the door, pull the chair out, guide the woman through a crowded venue and pay the bill at the end of the evening seems to be alien to most, if not all, modern men. Just remember behind every powerful man stands a great woman, so honour her and treat her with respect, even if you do just want to get in between her legs. I am not saying to act like a slave and treat the woman as if she is far superior to you but be gentle and show your humane side. After all, good manners and common courtesy don't cost a thing.

Speaking of cost, I want to speak briefly about covering the cost and who's responsibility it is. Ultimately, nobody owes anyone anything and the responsibility should lie with each individual. However, if you have asked the woman out on a date, then I think the responsibility should lie with you. After all, you are the one making the request to share her time, so I think it is only fair that you pay.

However, there is damage limitation regarding this, as follows: do not pick a place that will burn a hole in your pocket; do some research before asking the woman out on a date and if possible, make full use of Voucher Cloud app. There are often great deals on the Voucher Cloud app, so keep an eye out and make full use of it. Wowcher is another good one to use. This may seem extreme, but in the past, I have checked the food and drinks menu online, so that I have a rough idea of how much the evening will cost. It is always advisable to overestimate rather than underestimate the potential cost of the evening.

From a personal point of view, I find dinner dates far too formal, especially if you're meeting for the first time. I've always leaned towards taking a woman out for drinks, as I have found this a lot more relaxing and a lot less daunting. Moreover, I would much prefer it if a woman saw me spill a drink instead of seeing food stuck between my teeth. As the years have gone by, I have tended to leave the dinner dates to the 2nd or 3rd date, if of course I have got that far.

One thing that is a complete no and something that should be avoided, especially when going on a first date, is a trip to the cinema. When you're a teenage newbie to the world of dating, I think a trip to the cinema, in the hope you end up along the back row with your female companion is understandable, but as an Adult?? Hell no!!! Believe it or not some men still fall victim to this dating catastrophe and it comes as no surprise, when you spend 90 plus minutes sat in a darkened room, looking at the big screen in silence alongside a woman you've only just met, that it doesn't work out. Some may attempt to break the ice by taking the woman for a drink beforehand, but this invariably softens the devastating blow of disappointment. Be creative and don't be afraid to break away from the norm when going on the 1st or 2nd date. Ten pin bowling could be an option or a snazzy bar with ping pong tables. At the end of the day you want to stand out from the rest and appear as exciting and fun as possible, so don't be afraid to step out of your comfort zone and try something different. I can accept that there may be anxieties around choosing a place that doesn't meet expectations, but if a woman's decision not to see you again is purely based on the fact you chose a shit venue, then she really isn't worth worrying about.

CHAPTER 7 - CONNECTION IS KEY

During the dating process you will often hear women talk about chemistry and/or connection, and when I was a novice to the dating game, I thought it was this secret scientific formula regarding men and women, that only a select few were aware of. However, as time went by and I gained further experience, I learnt that they relate to two simple things: attraction and the way the woman interacts with you. Chemistry is all about attraction and is often a simplified way to describe that butterfly feeling a woman will feel when she meets a guy she's attracted to. That skipped heartbeat, sweaty palms and sensation of electricity passing through the veins are all related. You don't have to be a stud muffin to provoke such feelings within a woman. In fact, the physical element can be limited to something as small as a smile, or nice teeth, or nice eyes, or nice shaped lips. Either way there must be some form of attraction. The attraction could also be in the way you dress, the way you talk, the way you look at her, the list can go on and on.... Bottom line is, attraction does not always relate to physical appearance, and if it does you don't need to be picture perfect.

Connection is vital in the dating world and is important to note you cannot have chemistry without connection and vice versa. Connection relates to the woman's ability to communicate and interact with the man and is fundamental when it comes to obtaining and maintaining the woman's interest. Good thing is, you don't have to have a particular personality trait or be an outstanding communicator. All the woman seeks is a man who is willing and able to listen. Women like to feel heard and it is important that the woman feels as though you're present and taking on board all that she wishes to discuss. Women do not want solutions to issues they wish to talk about, nor do they want you to play devil's advocate, they just want you to simply listen. This might sound like an easy task but believe me there is nothing easy about actively listening, when somebody's 'chewing your ear off'.

I can remember a time back in 2011, when I was briefly dating a woman, and we were sat on the sofa at her place watching TV. I cannot remember for the life of me what we were watching, but she went into a 15-minute explanation of the problem she had with her eyes and reasons why she couldn't wear contact lenses. I had switched off after the first few seconds and paid absolutely no attention to a word she said, and this was clearly evident when I asked: "Why don't you just wear contact lenses?" She looked at me in complete shock and said "wow". I never saw her after that, and ever since then, I realised it is far better to give the impression you're listening, rather than not listen at all and get found out.

Therefore, if you are in a situation in which the woman clearly likes the sound of her own voice, simply say the following: "Is it?" "Really?" "Don't lie" "I hear you". Providing you use those phrases in order of relevance to what you are listening to, you don't have to listen to a single word she says, not unless you choose to of course. Ultimately, chemistry and connection are all to do with how you make the woman feel. As long as she feels like you're listening and she feels some attraction towards you, then you're certainly heading in the right direction in terms of your dating objectives, whatever they may be.

Communication is the only way to get your message across, no matter how big or small it may be. In fact, there are many ways in which we communicate in today's society, but despite the many innovative and creative ways available to us, body language still accounts for a large proportion of communication. According to Albert Mehrabian's Theory of Communication research study, 55% of communication is through body language, which is why I think it is paramount to pay close attention to the way the woman communicates, through her use of body language. With this in mind, try where possible to focus on the subtle clues she may not be consciously aware of. There are things we all do subconsciously, without giving them any real thought. For example, brushing our teeth, making the bed, drinking a cup of tea etc.... The things we do subconsciously are so embedded into the mind that there is no reason to consciously think of them. In other words, we do them automatically. In terms of the woman's body language, there are things she will convey without consciously knowing it, and it is here that you can capitalise and work out quite quickly whether or not she's interested in you. It is important to note here that I am not a body language expert, but there are things that I have observed, that have assisted me to ascertain whether the woman has interest in me or not. For example, the positioning of the woman's feet has always been a clear indicator as to whether or not she's interested in me. From my experience, the woman will be showing interest in me if one or both feet are pointing directly towards me. If she is unsure about me but there is some interest, one foot will be pointing away from me, while the other will point directly towards me. If, however both feet are pointing away from me then I would conclude that she isn't interested. Similarly, with the positioning of the woman's wrist. If her wrist is facing away from me but towards her, then it would suggest to me that she is guarded and does not feel completely comfortable. However, if her wrist is on display and facing towards me then this will suggest she feels at ease and comfortable within my company, but if her wrist is facing downwards towards the floor or table, then that would suggest to me she has absolutely no interest in me and is merely passing the time.

Some people say you can tell what a person is thinking through their facial expressions, and once upon a time I succumbed to this way of thinking, but this couldn't be further from the truth. In fact, facial expressions are perhaps the most misunderstood form of communication. For example, I was on a date about 6 months' ago, when the lady I was on a date with started talking about her love of Sushi. As she began to talk, I remembered that I had forgotten to defrost the chicken I had planned for my meal the following day. As this happened, the right upper corner of my lips pushed upwards as my eye brows formed a V shape, while simultaneously 'tutting' under my breath. I obviously pulled a facial expression of discontent, because she stopped mid-way and said "Oh maybe I better stop talking, because I'm talking way too much". This wasn't the case at all. I had just simply remembered what I had forgotten to do. So, while we may think we're experts at reading people's faces, most of the time we're way off the mark. Therefore, do not try to gauge what the woman is thinking by using her facial expressions as a guide.

When rounding off the date, a man would often hope for an invitation back to the lady's home to continue the evening, but this will not always be possible for reasons only the woman will know at the time. While some men will wallow within the depths of self-pity and view the date as a complete failure, others will patiently wait to see if they will get another crack at the whip. However, in order to save yourself the time and energy patiently waiting to know whether you'll see her again, you may be able to work it out quite quickly through her use of body language. For instance, when saying goodbye, the woman will subconsciously move towards you leading with her head going forward. She may tilt her head to one side to expose her cheek, but do not be too discouraged if she's not pouting her lips, as she moves closer, the exposure of her cheek could be a sign of her being shy and waiting for you to take the lead to have a kiss. However, if the woman remains still and you take the lead and go straight in for the kill (Kiss) and she turns at a slight angle and looks further away as she leans forward, then this is an indication that she isn't interested. She may in fact hug you, but the positioning of her head and the direction in which it goes could be a clear indicator.

CHAPTER 8 - TAKE CONTROL

There's a fine line between desire and desperation and it is essential for the man to be mindful of this. I say this because many men have made the fatal mistake of coming across as too keen, or in the woman's eye too desperate even though, according to the man, he is merely showing his interest/desire to get to know the woman. It is extremely tricky because if you show yourself to be too interested, or too available it's to your detriment, and if you show too little interest or availability the woman will simply look elsewhere. Therefore, I often use what I call 'mirroring' or reflective behaviour. For instance, if I text a woman and she respond's after 3 hours, I will take 3.5 to 4 hours to reply back to the text she responded to. I will always mirror the behaviour but alter it slightly, so it does not look too obvious or become too predictable. In addition to this I seldom text/call women over the weekend, because it can come across as though I have nothing better to do. I will, however make contact during the week between the hours of 8pm and 9pm. This is generally the time women unwind after a busy day at work or feeding and bathing the children. I prefer to leave two days in between contact, unless the woman contacts me first and I try not to respond immediately after contact has been made by the woman, although I do alter this so that a pattern does not develop. During the initial stages of contact, I will occasionally send the woman a morning text to wish them a good day. Some men may be reluctant to do this, as it may come across cheesy, but surprisingly, the women I have done this to have liked it because it shows that I have thought of them and I have held them in my mind. I do not make a habit of this and it is essential to keep contact sporadic and unpredictable. I can assure you from my experience this will get the woman hot on your heels. Again, you are not displaying behaviour she is accustomed to, or behaviour that is predictable, which feeds in to the concept of being hard to figure out, which as discussed moments ago works in your favour.

It is vitally important that you are patient. So many men, me included, have been reactive towards a woman who has not responded when she has been expected to do so. Our reaction to this is a direct result of the beautifully illustrated picture often created in our minds. So, if in the future a woman doesn't respond immediately to your call or text message, do not bombard her with further calls or text messages demanding an explanation as to why she has ignored you. The truth of the matter is she may not be ignoring you at all. In fact, she may have been caught up with something work-related, or she could have genuinely forgotten to get back in touch. I have been guilty of polluting my mind with thoughts of a woman deliberately ignoring me, but the basis for which this line of thinking formed, was from my own behaviour towards women I was not interested in, which often led to me ignoring them. Therefore, if I got ignored, I would assume (making an ASS out of U and ME) the woman was ignoring me, due to not being interested and would go on a rampage to get to the bottom of why I felt she had ignored me.

Women are like 'sniffer dogs' when it comes to desperation, and can sense if a man is desperate a mile off. If she catches a whiff of it, then it will prove to be the decisive blow in your pursuit to date her. Now we've all been subjected to moments of desperation, particularly when it comes to fulfilling our deepest needs and desires, but the key is how to manage that need/desire. I am not saying for one moment not to succumb to the feeling of desperation, but I am encouraging you to mask it. There are two instances in my own personal experience, in which I have done just that (masked it) and believe me the ordeal of having to do so was painful. The first instance happened back in 2010.

I had met this lady at Euston Station, she was obviously into fitness as her tight, navy-blue, polyester leggings clearly showed her well defined legs. Her vest was nicely cut to reveal her washboard stomach, which was complimented by her protruding oblique's. At the time I was desperate to date a woman who was into fitness, which was more to do with the novelty factor than anything else. Anyway, after a short chat, in which I convinced her that I was seeking some assistance with training and nutrition, we exchanged numbers. As soon as I got home, I texted her, and to my surprise she texted me the same evening, despite it being 2 hours' later. I was so overwhelmed with excitement, that I texted her back immediately and sent a further 2 more text messages, which did not get a response. I was left thinking that I had come across as too keen, which subsequently led me into thinking I had blown the opportunity to meet her, despite the fact it was all to do with fitness and nutrition. However, the following morning I received a text message from her apologising for not responding the night before. As a result of the text exchanges the night before, I held back with my response and took longer to reply. We eventually spoke on the phone and agreed to meet at a Café in Barnet to discuss a consultation. She quoted me £65.00 per hour for nutrition and training advice, which had me gasping for air. I was in a bit of a dilemma as I wasn't sure whether to come clean and tell her I wanted to get into her knickers, or go along with the whole thing in the hope she will one day pull them down voluntarily. After deliberating with myself I decided to come clean.

I called her and openly told her that I was not interested in training and nutrition, but before I finished, I could hear her chuckling. I was bemused as I had anticipated to be called every derogatory name under the sun, followed by her hanging up the phone, but to my amazement she said that she knew... We agreed to meet for a drink when time permitted. About a week had passed when I received a phone call asking me to come over. She was adamant nothing would happen between us and wanted me to come over to cheer her up, so I happily obliged. We spent the next couple of hours talking, drinking and chatting loads of shit. A few drinks and a couple of hours' later she stood opposite me, as I was seated on her dark red Chesterfield sofa, and she had a puzzled look on her face. I could feel my balls filling up, as my mind ran riot with all the things I was wanting to do to her, but I somehow managed to keep my composure. I distracted myself by asking why she had a confused look on her face? She said "I'm not used to this" and I replied "used to what?" she said "men just sitting there and not trying to jump on me. Normally by now a man would have tried it on me". In my head I was thinking "If only you knew..." but I kept my urge under wraps.

She looked like a fish out of water, completely lost and unsure of what to do. My actions were clearly a shock to her system, as well as my own, but I kept cool despite desperately wanting to pounce on her. I asked her to come and sit beside me and told her to relax and chill. As she sat down, she turned towards me and asked if she could kiss me? Just before I launched myself towards her, my inner being looked towards the heavens and blew a great big massive kiss, as I knew at that point my deepest desire to sleep with a fitness model was about to become a reality. I don't think there is any need to disclose what happened next, but by masking my inner desire, I was able to show her that I could maintain self-control and did not make me come across as desperate. This invariably attracted her towards me, and I made damn sure that I took full advantage of it.

The second instance happened sometime after that. I had arranged to meet a woman, whom I had spoken to on a dating website, at a coffee shop close to South Kensington. At the time I hadn't had sex in over 9 months and I was gagging for it. She was of a lean/muscular build, with silky dark brown hair and chestnut brown eyes. She had tattoos that covered her upper left shoulder and the lower right forearm. I can recall meeting her for the first time and wanting to tear her clothes off, but I managed to keep calm. During the date it turned out that she was very active in the 'Adult Industry' and this only added to my desperate need to fulfil my sexual desires. The more she spoke of her exploits within the Adult Industry, the more I began to think my chances to have my desires fulfilled would come to fruition. That was until she said "I never do anything on first dates". Considering she had come to London for a business trip and was due to travel back to Birmingham the next morning, I thought there was no chance of my ever getting my leg over this one, and that thought became even more apparent, when we left the coffee shop and said our goodbyes. Despite my need to have sex, as well as my strong physical attraction towards her, I accepted and respected her decision and the subsequent outcome of the date, even though I was crushed inside. The only consolation at that time, came when she leant over and gave me a nice tongue-filled kiss. I then left and made my way to the station. I remember thinking that it will be another evening on the Laptop scrolling through Pornhub and xHamster, but to my amazement I got a call on my phone just before I got to the escalators. It was her! She kindly asked me to return, followed by an invite back to her hotel room, which I happily accepted.

The key lessons I learnt from both instances, was the need to stay calm and conceal my desperate need to fulfil my sexual desire. Desperation in the eyes of many women is a sign of weakness and shows lack of control. By remaining calm and by not succumbing to your inner sexual demon, you illustrate self-control, which believe it or not is an attribute that can draw a woman towards you. There will be occasions where you won't be as lucky as I was on those two separate occasions, but that doesn't matter because some women have also mastered the art of self-discipline, which means if she doesn't succumb to her own inner sexual demon first time around, rest assure she may well do so, the next time you meet.

CHAPTER 9 - SEIZE THE MOMENT

Women have a tendency to think deeply, which can cause them to over analyse. This can work for you, but can also work against you, which is why I have adopted the 'strike while the iron is hot' principle. Women are experts at talking themselves into changing their minds, and their fickle nature, along with their ability to get lost within their own thoughts, makes 'striking while the iron is hot' fundamental, when attempting to seize an opportunity that presents itself. For example, I went on a date with a woman I met whilst working and every time I tried to arrange a second date, she was always too busy to meet. Suddenly, one evening after a hard, tiring and stressful day at work, she invited me over to her place for dinner. I was inclined to turn down the offer, due to feeling tired and stressed. Moreover, I had to work extremely early the following day. I had an internal dialogue and concluded that I may not get another opportunity like this again, so I seized the moment. The evening saw me open the passageway to many more invitations back to her place, but this may not have happened, had I not acted upon the opportunity that presented itself in the first place. Therefore, if a woman presents you with a chance, take it and do not procrastinate or think another opportunity will arise, because it may not happen and it is for this reason that you should always 'strike while the iron is hot'

One thing that can prove to be an Achilles' heel, is not having a place to go, after you have wooed the woman with your irresistible charm and charisma. Women, like men, have needs, and there are times when a woman will want that need to be fulfilled, so if you have laughed or charmed your way towards taking her to the bedroom, it is important that you have a place to take her afterwards. Believe it or not there are some men out there who still live at home with their parents, or those who think it is a bright idea to date women, whilst their spouse is at home. Either way, not having a place to take the woman, when it is clear she is willing to sexually engage with you, fucks you up every single time. Don't get me wrong, some may well resort to a Holiday Inn or Travel Lodge Hotel, but unless the woman you've met is a cheap whore, I would strongly suggest you don't do this.

Logistics, or the lack of it, is the one thing that has decimated opportunities that have come my way. Sad thing is, if you don't have a place to take the woman, when it is clear she is willing to spread her fluffy wings, then there really isn't much you can do. However, there are things you can do leading up to the date. The first thing you would need to establish is whether there is scope for any sexual engagement in the first place. Women can be quite blatant about this subject during the chatting/getting to know each other stage. So, if it reaches a point in which she's sending you pictures of her in her lingerie, or laying topless on her bed with her finger in her mouth, then you know there is a strong possibility something will go down. The next thing you should try to find out is whether there is a chance she is willing to take you back to her place? Again, during the chatting phase you could find out whom she lives with. Generally, from my experience it is highly unlikely that the woman will take you back to her home if her child or children still live at home, unless she sees you more as a long-term option. If the woman lives alone then the signs are definitely promising and if she has a flat mate/s then it most certainly isn't the end of the world.

When I have agreed to meet with a woman, I try to meet her as close to where she lives as possible. The reason I do this is because women, as discussed earlier, have a tendency to overthink, which can subsequently lead them towards changing their mind. Therefore, if we are at a bar or restaurant close to where she lives, and she does decide that she would like to explore more, then it leaves very little time for her to analyse the situation and question whether she is doing the right thing. As a result of this, it is important to keep the woman engaged in conversation and not to leave any time for her to go inside her head and start thinking.

If you are lucky enough to get an invitation back to the woman's home, do not assume that this is an easy access pass towards her vagina. Remember, to assume means you make an ASS out of U and ME! Also, it is always essential to remember that you approach any situation with women with an open mind, and without expectations. I say this because women, as mentioned earlier are sexual detectives and will try to find out as much as possible before deciding whether they want to go the full 9 yards. In addition, a woman will quickly try to figure out what your intentions are. As long as they coincide with her own, then whatever you intend to achieve will happen.

In the past, when I have made it beyond the threshold of the woman's home, I immediately go into a state of hyper-vigilance. I make sure that I scan as much as I possibly can within the first few seconds of entering the home. I do this for my own protection more than anything, but also to gauge the type of woman she may be. Generally speaking, you can get a pretty good idea of the woman and how she is as an individual, by the way she keeps her home. For example, through my experience I have found that women that are extremely clean and tidy tend to be very well organised and efficient. The way she keeps her place may not necessarily give me an indication of her skills within the bedroom, but at least I get a rough idea of whom I am involving myself with, in terms of hygiene and personality traits.

CHAPTER 10 - SELF INDULGE

I don't care how many books you read or how good you are at getting the attention of women, there are times when we all hit a dry spell. This can last weeks, months or in some rare cases even years, and believe me the dry spell can be painful. It is during this period that the self- esteem and confidence are put to the ultimate test, and while this period will provoke self -doubt, loss of confidence and frustration it is essential to maintain your identity and not allow your self- belief to be compromised. I accept that this is far easier said than done but remember the more you resist, the more it persists. So, if you find yourself in a situation in which you're being rejected by every female you approach, take this as a sign to spend more time with yourself and work on aspects that you wish to improve on. Personally, I have found it very useful to divert my attention away from women completely and focus it solely upon myself. I have found that by doing this, I become a better version of myself and I do not run the risk of falling victim to self -doubt. In addition to this, I inadvertently convert my mindset from one that is in a state of needing, towards a mindset that is in a state of wanting. Remember, Mother Earth provides each of us with all the things we need as human beings, anything else beyond that is extraneous. Therefore, the more you seek something you feel you need, which is beyond all that Mother Nature has provided for you, the more that thing you feel you need evades you. So, change the thought of needing into one of wanting and even if you are enduring a torrid time attempting to get a woman, try to adopt this line of thinking and it may just help you along the way.

Obviously, every man is different and while some of this may work for some, we cannot assume that it will work for all. Some men feed off female attention and will go to great lengths to achieve this. Therefore, the notion of diverting their attention away from the hand (women) that feeds their ego, is like dishing Superman a plate of Kryptonite. Subsequently, they tend to punch way below their weight in order to help boost their self-confidence, when they hit a dry spell. I have been guilty of this and have compromised my own self-worth to soothe a need, that really serves me no real long-term purpose. For example, during the height of my glory dating days I had 5 or more women on the go. Chatting, sleeping, eating and fucking different women as all part of a day to day routine. It became a full-time job, in which I needed a PA to organise my free time, as I would often double book myself and leave at least 2 of the 5 or more, women pissed off. The more I pissed them off, the more they became withdrawn, but I actually didn't give a shit, because I had plenty of others to occupy my time. Slowly but surely the numbers of women I had to occupy my time depleted one by one, until eventually I only had one or two. And by the time I was reduced to the couple I had, I managed to piss them off, because I now became too available and wanted to occupy too much of their time, which led them to ceasing contact. This then led to a dry spell, in which I had no women to occupy my time and then sought women that were below what I would go for, just to soothe my need (ego). While this was a short-term fix, it didn't serve any real purpose. I soon realised that I needed to focus on myself and give women less of my attention. Ironically, the less attention I gave women, the more they seemed to be interested. Before I knew it, women were coming out of the woodwork.

I think the hardest part within the dating game is to hold on to what you have, if you manage to get it. This could be the woman's attention, her interest in you, or the intimacy you have with each other. It's one thing acquiring something you want but it's another thing to maintain it, and with the ever-changing and ever-developing society we live in, people's ability to be patient or show tolerance is virtually non-existent. Which is why I believe it is far better for a woman to grow to like you, then it is for her to like you a lot at the beginning. Anything that doesn't grow or develop is dead. If a woman's liking for you reaches its peak, it can only go one way. Therefore, I believe it is important to leave room for her liking to grow, which is why some men use the 'be mean, keep her keen' approach.

If you take into account the relationships of our grandparent's generation, many of them were long lasting. Women and men alike were a lot more tolerant and far more persistent than they are these days. A man wouldn't give up after the 3rd knock back, let alone the 1st and there seemed to be an appreciation of that kind of mentality, but now if a man shows any kind of persistence, he's deemed a stalker, psychotic or weird. The irony of it is, women during their tender teenage years convey stalker like tendencies. Just ask any female you know how many posters they had up on their bedroom walls of their favourite popstar, or whether they knew all the latest news and gossip regarding their favourite popstar? I can guarantee you they could tell you virtually all you needed to know about their favourite pop idol, but yet a man shows some persistence and he's deemed a stalker? Don't get me wrong there are some proper fucked up people out there, stalkers included, but I do not think a man should be branded a stalker, if he is displaying a moderate level of persistence.

Persistence seems to be an infectious disease that everybody attempts to avoid. I mean why else has it eluded so many beings that live on this blue and green planet? The first sign of defeat and the man gives up. The first sign of a man annoying a woman and she replaces him with the next one. I think it is far too easy and far too accessible for people to simply 'hook up', that there appears to be little patience or value when we do actually meet. It's not until we feel like we've met someone who ticks most of the boxes we have presented, that we feel the need to take time and make a bit more effort. Sad but true, and this is the direction in which our society has taken us. So much so it is almost seen as a crime to take your time to get to know someone. I have lost count of the amount of times a woman has either ignored me or blocked me, because she felt we were spending far too much time talking. I mean since when was it a bad thing to talk to get to know someone? I remember one woman questioning whether I found her sexy, because I hadn't made any sexual advances during the two previous times we had met. I mean what the fuck???

Don't get me wrong, each to their own but the fun isn't in the acquiring of the prize but in the pursuit of it. I love the chase and I love pursuing the woman and doing all that I can to get her to give in and succumb to my way... I gain even more joy when the woman puts up some resistance and I end up getting her later. Persistence is a sign of resilience and the more you show in terms of those qualities, the more strength you obtain in terms of your character. I am not suggesting for one minute that you hound and pester any woman you wish to get with. No is no at the end of the day, and if it is clear she means no then simply move on. But I am talking about those times when you know you can have the woman and she's simply playing hard to get. In this case, a no does not necessarily mean a no and if it does then it's just for the time being.

CHAPTER 11 - PAY CLOSE ATTENTION

Once upon a time, most men would trip over their shoe laces in order to get between a woman's legs, while a woman would attempt to move heaven and earth in order to capture a man's heart. Although this is still very much the case, there has been some shift in what we generally seek in our sexual counterpart. Most women of today have been empowered into thinking they do not need a man, other than for reproduction purposes, while the increase in debauchery has left men wondering whether they will ever find a woman capable of keeping her legs closed. While the notion can evoke negative thoughts and feelings, men and women alike must remember: we are not friends, nor are we enemies but teachers. We each hold the reflective mirror for the other to see our flaws. Therefore, perceive each dating experience, and individuals you encounter, as a lesson. I believe through these encounters you begin to learn about the things you loathe, and the things you love about yourself.

    A good friend of mine could never quite understand why I spent so much time socialising with women I had met online, particularly when it was clear only one thing was on the agenda. He would often say "how do you manage to spend time with these chicks?" According to him, he hated the very thought of spending time with a woman, particularly when it came time for him to insert his penis into her- as he called it - "gaping hole". Whereas, for me the social aspect of any engagement I had with a woman was the aspect I liked most. Through these interactions, I learnt so much about each individual, but more importantly women as a whole. Some of the conversations I have had with women have been mind-blowing, and very insightful in terms of understanding how they think. Moreover, it enabled me to acknowledge aspects of myself I did not even consider to be a flaw or perceive to be an attribute; and to embrace the interaction as an enlightening experience. For example, a lady whom I was seeing for some time, shared her thoughts on something she heard from a man named T.D Jakes, that is Thomas Dexter Jakes Senior, a pastor, author and film maker in the USA.

According to TD Jakes there are 3 types of people who will come into your life. The first type of person he speaks of is a confidant. These are the people who are with you regardless, and will accept you just as you are, no matter what. When you are down in the dumps, they will be there with you, when you are elated and feeling on top of the world, they will be there with you. They will tell you about your strengths, but will not be afraid to get in your face and tell you about your flaws. These individuals will love you unconditionally and are rare to come by. You will be lucky if you have even one in your life time. The second type of person is a constituent; these people are not really into you but they are into what you are for. In other words, as long as you are into whatever they are into, they will be beside you, but the moment they meet somebody who can progress their agenda quicker, they will leave you in the blink of an eye, because they were never really into you, they were into what you were for. The third and last group of people are comrades; these people are neither into you nor into what you are for, however, they will join you to fight a common cause. Once this has been achieved, they will leave you because they were never into you, nor into what you are for.

Initially, after she told me this, I was a little dubious, mainly due to the fact it came from TD Jakes, who in my view is a bit of a Christian enthusiast, but the more I gave it thought, the more I came to realise how true and how relevant this is within the dating/relationship context. Think about it: if you meet a woman who is truly into you and accepts you for who you are, and she stays with you through thick and thin no matter what, then you can consider her to be a confidant. If a woman has a desire to have a family and that desire coincides with yours, then while you both share that common objective, she will stay with you. However, the moment it seems as though you are unable to provide her with that family she so desperately craves, then she will leave you, in which case she will be considered a constituent. Lastly, if a woman recently breaks up with a long-term partner and you meet her around the same time you break up with yours and there is physical attraction, it is likely that you will both try to heal and use each other as comfort to overcome the burden of hurt and disappointment. Once you have overcome the pain of the breakup, it is likely that you will each move on with your lives and go your separate ways (Comrade).

It was useful to take heed of that analogy, because it allowed me to navigate effectively through the dating scene. I began to acknowledge the type of women I was pursuing and I soon began to realise, that as long as I wanted to continue adding notches to my bed posts, I would only ever attract a woman who would seek the same at that time. A woman, as some of you may know, will take what she can get until she gets what she wants. So, until the moment the right man comes along, she will happily engage in meaningless casual sex. In other words, as long as our agenda coincides, we will be fucking each other until the cows come home, but the moment she finds what it is she truly desires (Mr Right), she will drop me like a hot cake, and it is for this reason I stopped getting pissed off after a woman decided she no longer wanted to see me after a couple of months. I accepted that she was nothing more than just a constituent (fuck).

In fact, many of the women you engage in casual sex with, are either constituents or comrades, so don't throw your toys out of the pram if she decides to leave you and perform a star jump onto some other dude's dick. After all, there is nothing meaningful or long term about casual sex and I have come to realise that the majority of women who like a fair bit, tend to be emotionally retarded. Not because they are too thick to gauge the concept of emotions, or the implications actions can have on them, but they are too emotionally damaged to take this on board. Most of the women I came across, who were self-proclaimed nymphomaniacs, were either emotionally and/or physically abused. Therefore, they detached themselves emotionally to prevent themselves from getting hurt. As a whole these women have insecurity issues, as well as low esteem. They use sex, and large amounts of it to fill a void, which is that of low self-worth. Don't get me wrong there are some women who just like cock, but from my experience, the ones who like it excessively tend to have deep rooted issues, but then again don't we all?

Had I taken the same viewpoint as my friend, there's a good chance I would not have been aware of what this lady had shared with me; and it is for this reason, I think it is important to make constructive use of your time whilst you're with a woman, and not see it as just a means to a sexual end. Don't get me wrong, there will be some women who will show no interest in you other than your submarine, which she hopes will be loaded with many sea men, but that does not mean the same line of thinking has to apply to you. In fact, I would suggest you use each dating experience and encounter as something to learn from, rather than simply something to get from, if that makes sense?

The same lady and I got into a debate about gender roles and why she felt it was a man's duty to always pay for a woman. According to her "men should always pay for the woman". As I mentioned earlier, I think the man should pay if he has asked to take the woman out. However, I do not believe the responsibility to pay should fall solely upon the man each and every time you decide to go out. This idea that men should always pay for a woman stems from the days a woman's place was in the kitchen, while the man went out to work. Women were seen and not heard within society and seldom had any rights to work. However, thanks to movements such as the Suffragettes', which gave women the right to vote, things have changed.

Women now have the right to work and earn a living the same as men do, so there should be no reason why a woman cannot contribute towards a night out, if it has been mutually arranged and agreed. I personally do not always look towards a woman to contribute, but if we have gone for a meal and I pay for the food and drinks, then the next time we go out I believe the food, or at the very least the drinks, should be paid for by the woman.

I appreciate that there are still inequalities, when it comes to pay between men and women within the working world but I wonder if women think of the same inequalities, when they gain free entrance into a night club before midnight, while the man has to pay £20 plus to get in? At the end of the day, most of us are caught up in the rat race, in which we all strive to keep our heads above water, so if a woman seeks to look after her own pocket, then why shouldn't you?

She also spoke about the need for a man to adapt to the needs of a woman, by compromising aspects of himself. I have no idea what planet this woman was from and it soon became clear, following her verbal diarrhoea, that we were not inhabitants of the same place, hence the eventual elbow; but it did raise some thought-provoking discussions, in which I concluded nobody should have to adapt to be with anyone. You should simply be and if you find yourself having to compromise aspects of yourself to soothe the needs of another, then that person isn't for you. Why should you alter yourself to fit into somebody else? If you want to listen to a particular radio station, then you have to get the right frequency to tune into that station, yes? So why should the interactions between men and women be any different? I believe this is a contributory factor as to why some women and men become resentful towards each other and eventually break up. "I don't know who I am anymore" is the classic line, when you spend time adapting to the needs of others, rather than simply being. It is no wonder, according to the longitude study carried out by Sociologist Michael Rosenfield that 70% of couples break up within the first year.

CHAPTER 12 - 'MAN UP'

What is masculinity and have the men of today lost sight of what it is to be masculine? One could be forgiven for thinking the latter, especially when so many men wear jeans tighter than women's leggings, or have a top that shows more of their chest, than a top would show a woman's cleavage. Moreover, the roles which we adopt and the concept of gender seem to be a lot more fluid these days. I don't think it is necessarily a bad thing but I do not think it's a great thing either.

While masculinity is not defined by a man's choice of clothing, it is defined by his attributes. For example, over here in the West masculinity is defined by attributes such as courage, assertiveness and independence. As discussed earlier, a lot of men are not courageous enough to make a move on a woman because they're afraid of being rejected, or what others might think of them if they get rejected. On a personal note I generally don't give a flying fuck. As far as I am concerned, the worst a woman could do is ignore me or tell me "No", neither of which are new found experiences and most people have experienced at least one or both. So, whilst the feeling of getting ignored or being told no isn't nice, those witness to it will have empathy. In other words, don't just be careless simply care-less about what people think.

It is useful to note that the greatest enemy to overcome is yourself. We can put so much negativity in the way we think of ourselves, or how we're perceived by others, that we can sabotage our own quest for happiness. The only opinion that really counts is the one you hold of yourself, unless it's that of someone who can greatly improve your physical, mental and emotional wellbeing. Therefore, why concern yourself with another person's opinion? After all, opinions do not equal fact and their perception is not a reflection of your reality. Thus, be more assertive. Being assertive doesn't mean being aggressive, it just means being self-assured and decisive. With the absence of concern regarding other people's opinion, you have the freedom to believe in yourself and effectively do the things you want to do rather than doing the things other people want you to do, namely women. Think about it...

While the acquisition of independence can have different connotations, I wanted to focus it towards self-governance. We are all different and we all possess different strengths and weaknesses. There will always be a person richer and poorer than you, better looking and not as good looking as you, some that will have more sex with women and others that will have less sex with women, than you. The point I am trying to make here is comparison is a pointless exercise. Don't try to model yourself on someone else or be somebody you're not. Embrace the person you are and work with you've got, and if there is an aspect of yourself you dislike then simply work on improving this area, if it's an area that can be worked on.

One of the most off-putting attributes a man can possess is insecurity. A man who is not sure of himself or confident within his own flesh is considered a weak man and women have zero tolerance for weak men. So, if you are on a date, or you're hand in hand with a woman you're dating, ditch the insecurity badge and embrace the fact the woman is with you. Boys will be boys and where possible will conduct a fair bit of window shopping (checking the lady out) as much as they can, but the onus isn't on the man looking at the woman, it is on the woman's responses towards it, but whatever the outcome always maintain your composure and never show yourself to be insecure. Even if you're quaking on the inside never show this.

I had a situation whilst on a date, in which a guy was hovering around our table. I knew in the back of his head he fancied his chances and probably thought 'what the hell is she doing with him?' It didn't faze me one little bit, because she was with me and not him, and even if she did entertain his advances, then I would know for sure that she wasn't the right person for me. There came a point when I needed to go toilet, and at first, I was very reluctant to go because I knew as soon as I left, he would try and make his move. However, the urge to go was too overwhelming so I went. Upon returning to the table there he was, stood over my date talking to her. She was smiling and was actively engaging in conversation. My immediate reaction was to go over and make my presence felt, but I held back and watched as it unfolded.

The sleazy greaseball cocksucker was in full flow when he suddenly got his phone out. It was at this point that my patience was really pushed, but I resumed my observation. My date was still smiling and actively talking to the guy, while he still had his phone in his hand. He then gestured to suggest she should give him her number but she shook her head. He gestured again and my date again shook her head. He had a nervous smile on his face and just before he was able to ask my date for a 3rd time I came along. My date looked relieved to see me and the guy looked bitterly disappointed. I simply smiled and asked: "Is everything ok?" As he withdrew himself from our table he said: "Yes mate, all good". I didn't utter a single word related to what I had observed and it wasn't until 30 minutes later that my date finally told me what had ensued. Most men would've reacted and gone in all guns blazing without actually seeing for themselves whether the woman they're with is a slithering snake, and while some women thrive on men fighting over them, these are generally the women who have attachment issues. Save the muscle for when it's really needed and never compromise your integrity. You are who you are and if the person you're with doesn't value you, or what you bring to the table, then simply move on.

Things are constantly in motion, in which we're part of the gradual process of change. Things are not what they were 70 to 80 years ago. Things are a lot more accessible and socially acceptable, which feeds into the instant gratification phenomena that has plagued western culture. We live within a 'here and now' mindset in which everyone is rushing to acquire whatever it is they desire. Amongst the chaos of us all trying to accomplish and experience the things we want, is a desperate need to reflect upon what is truly important. This is variable and unique to each individual but I had a heated debate with a group of male friends, who argued being with friends, family and focusing on money is important due to it being a constructive use of time. I argued that the concept of importance is unique to each individual and that we should not get bogged down with concerning ourselves with our perceptions of what we think/see as important, if it relates to someone else's perception of what they consider to be important. Don't get me wrong, it is vitally important to spend valuable time with friends, family etc... but to say that anything beyond that is a complete waste of time didn't quite sit right with me. People often talk about time as though there is never enough of it, but time by definition is the indefinite progress of existence. Therefore, why do we put such emphasis on the time we have and how much of it should be used and where, when we do not know exactly how much of it we have left? This then permeates through to people, thinking that certain things should be done by a certain time. For example, When I am aged 20, I must have a wife and kids, or when I am aged 30, I must own my own home. Everything then becomes time pressured.

I firmly believe that this has helped feed the YOLO (You Only Live Once) way of thinking and has led towards people seeking instant gratification, which then feeds into the whole revolving door experience within the dating world. 'If it isn't you, then it will be someone else' attitude is sending shock waves throughout the dating game, and this isn't just concerning to me within the dating context but within society as a whole. A man on a talk show stated that men and men alone have attributed towards the current situation, regarding men and women within modern day society, and have somehow led, through their behaviour towards the very reason why women have adopted a male like attitude. Once upon a time a woman's place was within the confines of her own home, while her man was supposed to be out working. While this was generally the case, it did not stop some men dipping their dicks somewhere else. As you are aware, women argue that this was seen as acceptable within the eyes of the general public. Fast forward to 2018, and women are seen as the perpetrators.

The man on the talk show argued that a man would often tell the woman what she wants to hear, in order to take what he wants. According to him this then led to many women being damaged. Later down the line a good man would come along hoping to heal the damaged woman, but he in turn gets hurt because of the pain she suffered. This then leads to the damaged man to go on and hurt a good woman and so on…. I couldn't help but agree with what the man was saying and while I accept men have played a major role in this, I do not think they are solely responsible. I guess the point of all of this is to highlight the fact that things are very different to how they once were and that women now are no longer seen as a cheap slag if they sleep with multiple men, and if they are seen that way, they certainly don't give a shit. Most things we see are sexualised and sex is no longer a taboo, it is everywhere and easily accessible. There are some who apply caution when discussing the topic of sex and some women who are conscious of the fact they can be seen as an easy target, but the issue isn't the topic of sex itself but how we and in particular men, go about getting it. There does not appear to be much class in the pursuit of anything these days, and if we do acquire something we have long desired, then there certainly doesn't appear to be much appreciation when we acquire it. Just remember, the acquisition of something is far easier than the maintenance of it. Therefore, if you do get the full attention of a woman, bear this in mind. After all, nothing lasts forever.

Acknowledgements

The publication of this book would not have been possible without Michael Terrence Publishing. A big thanks to Keith and Karolina at MTP. I would also like to thank Caroline Mylon for her assistance.

If it wasn't for James Scott, I probably would not have written this book, so a big thanks to you for planting that seed in my head, and of course a great big massive thanks to all of the women who have dated me, rejected me and accepted me. Without you, this would not have been possible.

I want to say a special thanks to Ray Austin as well as my Dad; who I sadly lost on the 24th August 2018.

I would like to extend my gratitude to anyone I have not mentioned. You know exactly who you are.

*Available worldwide from Amazon
and in all good bookstores*

----

www.mtp.agency

www.facebook.com/mtp.agency

@mtp_agency

www.ingramcontent.com/pod-product-compliance
Lightning Source LLC
LaVergne TN
LVHW041538060526
838200LV00037B/1035